chronic disease

Guide on chronic disease and how   to get rid off it

Dr Joe smith

Contents

chapter1

how it chronic disease
introduction to chronic disease

Chronic diseases refer to a group of medical conditions that are long-lasting, non-communicable, and often progressive in nature. These diseases have a significant impact on the health and well-being of individuals, families, and communities. Chronic diseases often develop slowly over time and can be caused by various factors such as genetics, lifestyle choices, and environmental factors. They include conditions such as diabetes, heart disease, cancer, stroke, and respiratory diseases. According to the World Health Organization (WHO), chronic diseases are the leading cause of death globally, accounting for 71% of all deaths worldwide. These diseases not only cause significant human suffering but also impose a heavy economic burden on individuals, healthcare systems, and society as a whole. The growing prevalence of chronic diseases has posed a major public health challenge, prompting the need for a deeper understanding of their causes, prevention, and management. One of the defining characteristics of chronic diseases is their long-term nature. Unlike acute illnesses that have a sudden onset and can be cured or managed within a relatively short period, chronic diseases persist for months or even years. They may require ongoing medical attention and can significantly impact an individual's quality of life. This long-term course of chronic diseases can lead to physical, psychological, and social consequences for patients and their families. The risk factors for chronic diseases are diverse and interrelated, making their prevention and management a complex and challenging task. Some of the common risk factors include unhealthy diets, physical inactivity, tobacco use, excessive alcohol consumption, and environmental factors such as air pollution. Additionally, genetics and other underlying medical conditions can also increase an individual's susceptibility to chronic diseases. One of the most concerning aspects of chronic diseases is their rising prevalence. The WHO reports that the global burden of chronic diseases is expected to increase by 57% in the coming decades. This is attributed to the rapidly aging population, unhealthy lifestyles, and inadequate access to healthcare in many parts of the world. As chronic diseases become more prevalent and complex, they require a multidisciplinary approach involving healthcare providers, policymakers, and individuals to effectively address the growing burden. The impact of chronic diseases is not limited to individual health but also extends to economic and social aspects. Chronic diseases can cause significant financial strain on individuals and their families due to the high costs of long-term treatment, medication, and care. They can also lead to decreased productivity, early retirement, and loss of employment, resulting in a ripple effect on the economy. Therefore, addressing chronic diseases is not just a health concern but also a socio-economic imperative. Despite the challenges posed by chronic diseases, there is growing evidence that many of them are preventable through lifestyle modifications and early detection. This has led to the concept of "prevention is better than cure" and the promotion of healthy living behaviors as a crucial strategy in reducing the burden of chronic diseases. By adopting a healthy diet, engaging in regular physical activity, avoiding tobacco and excessive alcohol use, and managing stress levels, individuals can significantly reduce their risk of developing chronic diseases. Moreover, effective management of chronic diseases is essential in improving the quality of life for individuals living with these conditions. This involves a comprehensive and collaborative approach that includes regular monitoring, timely treatment interventions, and self-management practices. Healthcare providers play a critical role in managing chronic diseases, providing patients with education, support, and necessary resources for proper disease management. In recent years, health systems and policymakers have recognized the urgency of addressing chronic diseases and have implemented various initiatives and policies to tackle them. These include promoting healthy lifestyles, increasing access to quality healthcare, implementing effective disease prevention and management programs, and conducting research to better understand the complex nature of chronic diseases. Governments and international organizations have also taken steps to address chronic diseases at a global level, with the adoption of the Sustainable Development Goals that include reducing the burden of non-communicable diseases. In conclusion, chronic diseases are a significant public health challenge that requires an integrated and multi-pronged approach to address. With their long-term impact on individuals, families, and communities, it is crucial to focus on prevention, early detection, and effective management to reduce the burden of these diseases. By promoting healthy lifestyles, ensuring access to quality healthcare, and implementing effective policies and programs, we can work towards creating a healthier and more sustainable future for all.

chronic disease list

Chronic diseases are responsible for approximately 70% of global deaths, making them a major public health concern. They not only cause a significant burden on individuals but also on healthcare systems and economies around the world. There are a multitude of chronic diseases, and they can affect any part of the body.

However, some of the most common chronic diseases include heart disease, diabetes, cancer, chronic respiratory diseases, and mental health disorders. Heart disease, also known as cardiovascular disease, refers to a range of conditions that affect the heart, such as coronary artery disease, arrhythmia, and heart failure. It is the leading cause of death globally, accounting for over 17 million deaths every year. Risk factors for heart disease include high blood pressure, high cholesterol, obesity, tobacco use, and a sedentary lifestyle. These risk factors can be managed and reduced through healthy lifestyle choices, such as regular exercise, a balanced diet, and avoiding tobacco use. Diabetes is a chronic disease that occurs when the body is unable to produce enough insulin or use it effectively, resulting in high blood sugar levels. There are two main types of diabetes: type 1 and type 2. Type 1 diabetes is autoimmune and often diagnosed in childhood, while type 2 diabetes is more common in adults and is often associated with obesity and sedentary lifestyle. If left unmanaged, diabetes can lead to serious complications, such as heart disease, kidney disease, nerve damage, and blindness. Regular monitoring of blood sugar levels, following a healthy diet, and engaging in physical activity are essential for managing diabetes. Cancer is a broad term used to describe a group of diseases characterized by uncontrolled cell growth. There are many different types of cancer, and they can occur in any part of the body. Some of the most common types of cancer include lung, breast, and colorectal cancer. The risk of developing cancer is influenced by various factors, such as genetics, environmental factors, and lifestyle choices. Early detection through screening tests and adopting healthy behaviors, such as avoiding tobacco use and maintaining a healthy weight, can help prevent or manage cancer. Chronic respiratory diseases are conditions that affect the lungs and airways, such as asthma, chronic obstructive pulmonary disease (COPD), and cystic fibrosis. These conditions make breathing difficult and can lead to serious complications, including respiratory failure. Asthma is the most common chronic respiratory disease, affecting over 339 million people worldwide. Although there is no cure for chronic respiratory diseases, symptoms can be managed through medication, inhalers, and avoiding triggers, such as air pollution and tobacco smoke. Mental health disorders, such as depression, anxiety, and bipolar disorder, are also considered chronic diseases. These conditions affect a person's thoughts, emotions, and behavior and can significantly impact their daily lives. Globally, over 264 million people live with depression and over 300 million people live with anxiety disorders. Mental health disorders can be caused by a combination of genetic, environmental, and social factors. Treatment for mental health disorders typically involves a combination of medication, therapy, and lifestyle changes. Although each of these chronic diseases has its own unique characteristics, they share many common risk factors and can often be prevented or managed with similar lifestyle changes. Adopting a healthy lifestyle, including eating a balanced diet, engaging in regular physical activity, avoiding tobacco and excessive alcohol consumption, and managing stress, can help prevent the development of chronic diseases. It is also crucial to get regular check-ups and screenings to identify any potential health issues early on. The burden of chronic disease goes beyond individual health concerns and has a significant impact on healthcare systems and economies. Chronic diseases account for a large proportion of healthcare spending, and the costs are expected to rise as the global population ages. In addition, chronic diseases can affect a person's ability to work and lead to productivity losses, further adding to the economic burden. In many parts of the world, there are significant disparities in access to healthcare and resources for preventing and managing chronic diseases. Lower-income countries often have a higher prevalence of chronic diseases and less access to resources for prevention and treatment, leading to a greater burden on already strained healthcare systems. Efforts to address chronic diseases must include a combination of individual-level interventions, such as lifestyle changes and screenings, as well as systemic changes, such as improved access to healthcare and education. Prevention and early detection strategies should also be prioritized to reduce the burden of chronic diseases and improve overall health outcomes.

chapter2

how to prevent chronic disease

1. Eat a Healthy and Balanced Diet One of the key factors in preventing chronic diseases is maintaining a healthy and balanced diet. This means incorporating a variety of fruits, vegetables, whole grains, lean proteins, and healthy fats into your daily meals. Avoid processed and high-sugar foods, as they can increase the risk of developing chronic diseases such as diabetes, heart disease, and obesity. Additionally, limit your intake of red and processed meats, as they have been linked to an increased risk of certain cancers. By following a healthy and balanced diet, you can provide your body with the necessary nutrients to function properly and

reduce the risk of chronic diseases. 2. Engage in Regular Physical Activity Regular physical activity is essential for maintaining good overall health and preventing chronic diseases. It can help improve cardiovascular health, strengthen bones and muscles, and reduce the risk of obesity, diabetes, and high blood pressure. Aim for at least 30 minutes of moderate-intensity exercise, such as brisk walking, cycling, or swimming, five times a week. If you have a sedentary job, make sure to get up and move around every hour to prevent prolonged sitting, which has been linked to increased risk of chronic diseases. 3. Avoid Smoking and Limit Alcohol Consumption Smoking is one of the leading causes of preventable death worldwide. It not only increases the risk of lung cancer and respiratory diseases but also contributes to heart disease, stroke, and other chronic conditions. If you are a smoker, quitting is the best thing you can do for your health. Additionally, limiting alcohol consumption is also important in preventing chronic diseases. Excessive alcohol consumption has been linked to liver disease, heart problems, and some types of cancer. If you choose to drink, make sure to do so in moderation, which is no more than one drink per day for women and two drinks per day for men. 4. Get Regular Health Screenings Many chronic diseases are asymptomatic in their early stages, making regular health screenings essential for early detection and treatment. Consult with your healthcare provider and get regular check-ups, screenings, and vaccinations based on your age, family history, and other risk factors. Some common health screenings include blood pressure, cholesterol, blood sugar, and cancer screenings. By identifying any potential issues early on, you can prevent chronic diseases or manage them more effectively. 5. Manage Stress Stress can have a negative impact on our physical and mental health, increasing the risk of chronic diseases such as heart disease, obesity, depression, and anxiety. Therefore, it is important to find healthy ways to manage stress, such as exercise, meditation, deep breathing, or talking to a therapist. Knowing your triggers and finding coping mechanisms can help reduce stress levels and improve overall well-being. 6. Practice Good Hygiene Practicing good hygiene can prevent the spread of germs and reduce the risk of chronic infections. Wash your hands frequently with soap and water, especially before and after handling food, after using the bathroom, and after coughing or sneezing. Cover your mouth and nose with a tissue when sneezing or coughing and avoid sharing personal items, such as towels or utensils, with others. These simple actions can help prevent the spread of diseases and keep you healthy. 7. Maintain a Healthy Weight Obesity is a major risk factor for many chronic diseases, including heart disease, diabetes, and some types of cancer. Therefore, it is essential to maintain a healthy weight through a combination of a healthy diet and regular physical activity. If you are overweight or obese, consult with your healthcare provider for a weight loss plan that is safe and effective for you. 8. Get Enough Sleep Getting enough quality sleep is crucial for maintaining good health and preventing chronic diseases. Lack of sleep can weaken the immune system and increase the risk of chronic diseases such as diabetes, heart disease, and obesity. Most adults require 7-9 hours of sleep per night. To improve sleep quality, establish a regular sleep schedule, create a comfortable sleep environment, and avoid electronics before bedtime. 9. Limit Exposure to

Environmental Toxins Exposure to environmental toxins such as air pollution, pesticides, and chemicals can increase the risk of chronic diseases. Limit your exposure to these toxins by using natural cleaning products, avoiding areas with heavy pollution, and eating organic food. If you work in a toxic environment, take necessary precautions to protect yourself. 10. Stay Socially Connected Having a strong social support system is important for both physical and mental health. Studies have shown that people who are socially isolated are at a higher risk of developing chronic diseases. Make an effort to stay connected with family and friends, join community groups or clubs, and volunteer in your community.

Having a support system can help reduce stress levels and improve overall well-being

chronic disease management

The key to managing chronic diseases lies in addressing the underlying risk factors that contribute to their development. These risk factors can be behavioral, environmental, or genetic. For instance, smoking, physical inactivity, unhealthy diet, and excessive alcohol consumption are major behavioral risk factors for chronic diseases. Exposure to air pollution, second-hand smoke, and chemicals are environmental risk factors. Genetic factors play a role in diseases such as diabetes, heart disease, and some types of cancer. Therefore, an integrated approach that addresses all these risk factors is crucial for effective management and prevention of chronic diseases. The first step in managing chronic diseases is accurate diagnosis and monitoring. Medical professionals use a range of tools and tests to diagnose chronic diseases and assess their severity. This may include blood tests, imaging tests, and screening procedures. Once a diagnosis is confirmed, regular monitoring is necessary to track the progression of the disease and adjust treatment accordingly. A key component of chronic disease management is self-care. This involves empowering individuals with the necessary knowledge and skills to manage their condition and prevent its complications. Self-care involves making lifestyle changes such as quitting smoking, adopting a healthy diet, and engaging in regular physical activity. It also includes learning how to manage symptoms, adhere to medication regimens, and recognize warning signs of complications. With proper self-care, individuals can play an active role in controlling their disease and improving their overall health. Another important aspect of chronic disease management is medication and treatment. Most chronic diseases require long-term medication to control symptoms, prevent complications and slow disease progression. These medications can include drugs to manage blood sugar levels, blood pressure, cholesterol, and other conditions. Treatment options may also include surgeries, procedures, and therapies such as chemotherapy or radiation for cancer. Medical professionals work closely with patients to develop individualized treatment plans that best suit their needs and preferences. In addition to medical management, a supportive healthcare team is essential for the effective management of chronic diseases. This team may include physicians, nurses, dietitians, pharmacists, and other healthcare professionals who work together to provide comprehensive care. The role of the healthcare team may extend beyond the treatment of symptoms and may also involve counseling and education to help individuals cope with the emotional and psychological impact of living with a chronic disease. Technology has also played a significant role in enhancing chronic disease management. With the advent of electronic health records, medical professionals have access to patients' medical history, test results, and treatment plans, allowing for more efficient and coordinated care. Patients can also use technology to track their symptoms, monitor their diet and activity levels, and communicate with their healthcare team remotely. This can improve treatment adherence and provide timely interventions to prevent disease complications. Managing chronic diseases also requires addressing the social determinants of health. These are the economic, social, and environmental factors that contribute to health disparities and impact the health of individuals and communities. For instance, poverty, limited access to healthcare, and inadequate education can hinder an individual's ability to manage a chronic disease effectively. Addressing these underlying factors is crucial for improving overall health outcomes and reducing the burden of chronic diseases. Moreover, prevention plays a significant role in chronic disease management. As the saying goes, "prevention is better than cure," and this is especially true for chronic diseases. Preventive measures such as regular health screenings, immunizations, and health education can help identify and manage risk factors early on and prevent the development of chronic diseases. Governments and healthcare systems must also prioritize public health policies and initiatives that promote healthy behaviors and reduce the burden of chronic diseases.

chapter3
causes of chronic disease

There are various factors that can contribute to the development of chronic diseases. These include both genetic and environmental factors. In this essay, we will explore the various causes of chronic diseases and how they can be addressed. 1. Genetics Genetics plays a significant role in the development of chronic diseases. Certain genes can make individuals more susceptible to conditions such as cancer and diabetes. While genetics cannot be changed, understanding a person's genetic predisposition can be crucial in identifying specific risk factors and taking preventive measures. For instance, individuals with a family history of heart disease can make lifestyle changes to lower their risk, such as exercising regularly and eating a healthy diet. 2. Unhealthy Lifestyle Habits Unhealthy lifestyle habits, particularly poor diet and lack of physical activity, are significant contributors to chronic disease. A diet high in saturated fats, sugars, and processed foods increases the risk of developing conditions such as heart disease, diabetes, and obesity. Sedentary lifestyles, due to long working hours and modern devices, have also contributed to an increase in chronic diseases. Regular exercise not only helps in maintaining a healthy weight but also reduces the risk of developing chronic conditions. 3. Tobacco Use Tobacco use is one of the leading causes of preventable chronic diseases, such as lung cancer and heart disease. Cigarette smoke contains thousands of chemicals, many of which are carcinogenic and can damage cells in the body. Smoking also increases the risk of developing respiratory diseases such as chronic bronchitis and emphysema. Second-hand smoke can also cause chronic diseases, making it harmful not only for smokers but also for those around them.

4. Excessive Alcohol Consumption

Excessive alcohol consumption is another cause of chronic diseases. Alcohol abuse has been linked to various health problems such as liver and kidney disease, heart disease, and several types of cancer. Heavy drinking can weaken the immune system, making individuals more susceptible to infections and diseases. Responsible alcohol consumption and avoiding binge drinking can help prevent the development of chronic diseases. 5. Environmental Factors Environmental factors such as air and water pollution, exposure to toxic chemicals, and radiation can also contribute to chronic diseases. Air pollution, for example, has been linked to respiratory diseases such as asthma and chronic obstructive pulmonary disease (COPD), while water pollution has been linked to increased cancer risk. Exposure to harmful chemicals in the workplace or household products can also have long-term health effects. 6. Stress Chronic stress can lead to a weakened immune system, putting individuals at a higher risk of developing various chronic diseases. High levels of stress hormones such as cortisol can increase blood pressure, heart rate, and constrict blood vessels, which can contribute to heart disease. Stress can also lead to unhealthy habits such as overeating, excessive alcohol consumption, or smoking, which can further increase the risk of chronic diseases. 7. Aging As individuals age, they become more susceptible to chronic diseases. Aging causes changes in the body, such as a decrease in muscle mass and an increase in body fat. These changes can lead to conditions such as heart disease, diabetes, and osteoporosis. As the body ages, it also becomes less able to fight off infections and diseases, making older adults more vulnerable to chronic conditions. 8. Poor Access to Health Care Lack of access to quality health care can also contribute to the development of chronic diseases. Individuals who do not have regular check-ups or do not seek medical help when needed are at a higher risk of developing chronic conditions. People living in rural areas or low-income areas may have limited access to health care services, making it challenging to manage and treat chronic diseases effectively. 9. Infectious Diseases Some chronic diseases can be caused by infectious diseases, such as HIV/AIDS and hepatitis B or C. These infections can damage vital organs, leading to conditions such as liver disease, kidney disease, and cancer. Vaccines and other preventive measures can help prevent these infectious diseases and reduce the risk of developing associated chronic diseases.

The end

www.ingramcontent.com/pod-product-compliance
Lightning Source LLC
Chambersburg PA
CBHW051925250726
48659CB00002B/850